CONTENTS

Written and edited by Jim Pollard • Cartoons by John Byrne.

Special thanks to Gambling With Lives and Gamblers Anonymous for their assistance with the development of this booklet. Thanks also to all the men who supported us by suggesting questions and sharing their stories. Some names have been changed.

Men's Health Forum advisory team: Dr John Chisholm, Dr Su Wang, Sara Richards and Ruth Pott.

First published: June 2023 · Next revision: June 2026

86% of gross online betting profits come from 5% of customers. You do the maths.

INTRODUCTION

How can gambling be a health problem? Our screens are full of gambling adverts. Actors, sports players and football managers… They wouldn't do it if gambling was so unhealthy. It wouldn't be legal.

Any of that sound familiar? Gambling does seem to be everywhere. This makes it appear very normal. And, in a way, it is. Gambling has been around as long as we have. But that doesn't mean it's harmless.

The thing is that, once upon a time, anyone who was anyone promoted smoking - the biggest celebs like Frank Sinatra and Joan Crawford, the greatest sports stars like Stanley Matthews, Joe Louis and Joe DiMaggio, even Laurel and Hardy. The list is endless.

But it doesn't happen anymore. Everyone knows smoking can kill. Cigarette packets carry public health warnings and advertising is banned.

But it took a long time and a lot of deaths to get to this stage. As recently as 1994, over forty years after the first research pointing to the harm caused by smoking was published, tobacco industry executives stood up in the US Congress and, one after the other, denied that nicotine was addictive. They knew they were not telling the truth.

This is roughly where we are with gambling now. There's plenty of research and evidence pointing to the dangers but the industry and the regulators haven't caught up.

As well as the serious health risks, the risk of running up ruinous debt makes gambling one of the most dangerous of addictions. One study suggested that people with a gambling disorder are 15 times more likely to take their own lives than the population in general.

The risk of developing a gambling disorder has increased with online gambling. This manual looks at why that is. It will help you to spot the warning signs of gambling disorder. That way, armed with the facts rather than celebrity endorsements, you can make your own decisions about whether and how you want to gamble and get support if you need it.

HOW GAMBLING WORKS

Whether it's betting on the toss of a coin, a football match or a hand of cards, gambling involves risking something of value (usually money) on guessing or predicting something that will happen in the future.

IS IT JUST LUCK?

Because you're predicting the future there is always some luck involved. Some forms of gambling involve nothing but luck such as the National Lottery, a scratch-card or a spin of a roulette wheel. The numbers that come up and whether they are winners is down to pure chance.

The chances of winning the National Lottery are now one in 45 million. In other words, you need to be very lucky indeed. For comparison, bookmakers will usually quote the odds of aliens landing on Earth as 100,000-1!

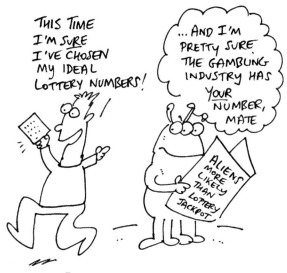

Other forms of gambling involve an element of skill or knowledge. You might increase your chance of winning your bet on a football match if you know who's playing. The past performances of the team and the players might give you a clue as to what will happen in the future. Same for horse-racing and most other sports betting.

Betting usually involves putting up a stake - a fixed amount of money which you will lose if you lose and get back if you win. But some forms of betting such as spread betting can see you lose more and more multiples of your stake, the more and more wrong you are with your prediction of the future.

HOW DOES THE INDUSTRY MAKE ITS MONEY?

Bookmakers make their money by ensuring the odds they offer are always slightly in their favour. If you do the maths on the odds bookmakers offer on, say a football match, you'll see they don't quite add up. The odds on the three possible outcomes (home win, away win and draw) always add up to over 100%. That is to say, the likelihood of each outcome is slightly over-estimated. That extra is the bookie's margin.

Casinos make their money through what's sometimes called the house edge. The easiest way to understand all this is to think of the roulette wheel. As the wheel is numbered from one to 36, the odds on your chosen number coming up should be 35-1. But in fact, there is also a zero (or sometimes a double or triple zero) putting the real odds higher. When the zero comes up, the house - the casino - wins.

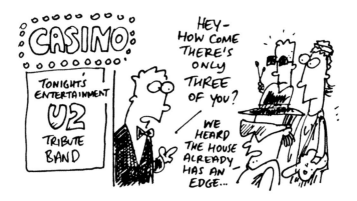

I DON'T UNDERSTAND ODDS, STAKES AND SO ON.

If you're interested in gambling but don't understand the maths (or anything else in this booklet), it makes sense to find out more. You wouldn't play a sport without knowing the rules.

HOW MUCH DOES THE GAMBLING INDUSTRY MAKE?

The UK gambling industry is enormous. According to the Gambling Commission, it made over £14 billion gross profit in 2020-21. The UK is the world's largest regulated online gambling market - outstripping even the USA. A House of Lords report from 2020 put gambling industry spending on advertising at £1.5 billion. So the best bet is probably a job in the industry!

DON'T SOME MAKE A LIVING FROM GAMBLING?

It's not unknown for people who have plenty of money to start with to make a little more through gambling. But it's rare. Indeed, with online gambling, winning accounts are often restricted, closed or frozen.

Think of it this way: the gambling industry needs to pay for all those glossy ads, sponsorships and promos, all those outlets, shops and sites, all those salaries and share dividends, plus pay the winnings of a few 'professional' gamblers and make a nice, tidy profit on top. Where does all that dosh come from? From one place only: the vast majority who mostly lose.

If you think you know a bit about gambling, do the maths. The odds on being a successful professional gambler may not be as long as on winning the National Lottery, but they're heading in that direction.

ALWAYS A LOTTERY

You may hear that you can boost your lottery chances by, for example, choosing less popular numbers. But this only improves your chances of not sharing the jackpot if you do win. It doesn't increase the chances of the numbers coming up. Nor does the fact that a number has come up a lot in the past increase or decrease its chances of coming up in the future.

BUT SOME LOTTERIES GIVE TO GOOD CAUSES.

True. Some gambling ads seduce you with big name stars, others with 'good causes'. But it's worth checking what percentage actually goes to 'good causes' - it's generally less than a third. If you want to support a particular charity or cause, it's better to give directly.

I GET ALL THAT, BUT GAMBLING IS EXCITING.

That's down to dopamine, a neurotransmitter first identified in 1957. It's the brain chemical that prompts us to do things we enjoy. We get a boost of dopamine when doing what we enjoy and also in anticipation of doing it.

It's understandable that we feel excited when we win. But because you get a thrill in anticipation of the next bet, you can also get a buzz when you lose. This means it can become very difficult to know when to stop. Some gamblers even say the buzz from losing is in some ways stronger than from winning because then you have the thrill of the chase.

MAYBE, BUT I'VE GOT THE KNACK.

An early big win is part of many stories of addiction. If you do well early on in your gambling career, it is possible to forget that all you are doing is guessing the future. It is easy to think you have a knack or some special skill or knowledge or data set that gives you an 'edge'.

This is incredibly seductive for some of us (nearly as seductive as the dopamine hits themselves). But take a step back and you can see that it is false. It's magical thinking. Nobody knows the future and however much research you put into your bet, whether it comes off or not will always be a matter of chance and can never be anything else.

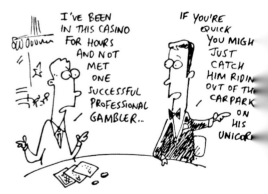

WHAT ARE GAMBLING HARMS?

The annual survey for the charity GambleAware found one gambler in eight was at some risk from their gambling. Other studies suggest it could be even more - perhaps one in four. The majority of these are men.

HOW MANY ARE AT SERIOUS RISK?

GambleAware reckon about 2.8% of all gamblers are at high risk. This adds up to more than one-and-a-half million adults in the UK.

These risk levels are assessed using something called the Problem Gambling Severity Index (PGSI). The PGSI is based on asking gamblers the sort of questions you'll find on page 12. If you have a score of 3 or more you're at moderate risk, a score of 8 or more and you're at high risk and in that group of 1.5 million. Even those at moderate risk are showing signs of addictive behaviour.

Gambling harms don't just affect the gambler. About 6% of the adult population are negatively affected by another's gambling.

WHAT SORT OF PROBLEMS?

The Mental Health Foundation say gambling can cause low self-esteem, stress, anxiety and depression. The gambling itself and the lying and cheating that addiction leads to can destroy relationships, families and lives. Some wind up homeless or in prison. (About a quarter of all prisoners have a gambling problem.) Gambling can take everything you have - not just money.

The Office for Health Improvement and Disparities reckons there could be near to 500 gambling-related suicides a year in England. Factor in Scotland, Wales and Northern Ireland and we're getting close to 600 gambling-related suicides a year in the UK.

ARE SOME TYPES OF GAMBLING MORE DANGEROUS?

Yes, if your only flutter is a weekly National Lottery ticket, you're probably reasonably safe. More dangerous forms of gambling include online slots, fixed-odds betting terminals (FOBTs) and 'in-play' sports betting where bets can be placed quickly and frequently. The speed intensifies the behaviour, so you're in a bubble of dopamine-fuelled delusion.

A Gambling Commission report found a 45% addiction rate with online slots, meaning that nearly half of the people who start to play will be negatively affected. 'In play' (micro-betting) gamblers are at even higher risk - 78% meet the criteria for problem gambling.

ONLINE GAMBLING IS MORE DANGEROUS?

Yes. You can bet very quickly and, perhaps most importantly, the apps and sites are deliberately designed to encourage you to do this. Based on your previous behaviour, the apps' algorithms know what you like and keep giving you a little bit more. Of course, all apps on our phone do this. But it's one thing to spend too long on social media, it's quite another to gamble all your money away.

When you keep having too much of a good thing, the brain's self-regulatory mechanism (called homeostasis) gives you diminishing returns. You need more of whatever it is to get the same high and indeed the high seems to get further and further away. Anyone who has ever binged on a bar of chocolate knows this. The first square tastes divine. The last three you wolf in one go and hardly notice.

The point is that this is exactly what is going on every time you click online on whatever it is you're interested in. In the case of gambling there's also money in the mix. A very heady - and dangerous - combination.

Some supposed financial trading apps, especially those that use gaming imagery like tumbling confetti and 'leaderboards' to attract 'investors', are also risky. The Financial Conduct Authority reckon that one in five users of such apps are at risk of problem gambling using the PGSI. Indeed, one gambling blocker app Gamban has now added trading apps to its banned list.

DOESN'T THAT MEAN EVERYONE IS AT RISK?

The smartphone and other tech allow us to gamble whenever and wherever we want to - all day, every day, if we wish.

Pretty much anyone can become addicted. The way online gambling works increases the risk for all of us.

IS THERE ANYTHING THAT INCREASES YOUR RISK?

Being male and being young. Compulsive gambling is more common in men than women and, the younger you start, the greater the risk of developing a problem.

Some health problems including depression, anxiety, bipolar disorder, obsessive-compulsive disorder (OCD) or attention-deficit/hyperactivity disorder (ADHD) might increase the risk. (Although some might argue that it's the other way round: compulsive gambling causes mental health problems.)

There is a class of prescription drugs called dopamine agonists used in conditions such as Parkinson's disease and restless legs syndrome. As the name implies, they affect dopamine levels and can increase compulsive behaviour including gambling.

Gambling disorder is also more common if you have friends or family who also have it, if you're highly competitive or if you engage in other compulsive behaviours such as smoking, drinking or working excessively.

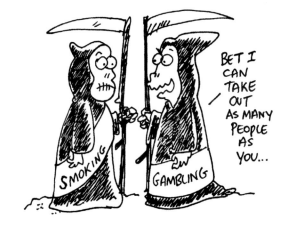

HOW DO I KNOW IF I HAVE A PROBLEM?

If you find yourself compulsively playing games of pure chance such as scratch-cards or online spins, you should, theoretically, quickly realise that you have a problem. After all, logic, as you've read in this booklet, tells you that you can't win in the long run. The trouble is the dopamine hits tell you different.

The chances of not recognising you have a problem are even higher when your gambling involves some degree of skill. Not only is the dopamine encouraging you to keep going but so is the part of you that tells you that you know a lot more than the other punters about football or horses or poker or whatever.

Don't fall for the old myths. Just because you can afford to lose (at the moment) or aren't playing every day (yet), doesn't mean you haven't got a problem.

Ask yourself honestly how you're feeling. Are you feeling anxious, down or depressed? Are you stressed, irritable or not sleeping well? Does your mood swing? Do you feel disconnected from the people and situations? All these could suggest your gambling is having an impact on your wellbeing.

This is the questionnaire the NHS suggests to help you assess whether gambling is becoming a problem. It is very similar to the PGSI mentioned on page 9.

> Do you bet **more than you can afford** to lose?

> Do you need to gamble with **larger amounts** of money to get the same feeling?

> Have you tried to win back money you have lost (**chasing losses**)?

> Have you **borrowed money or sold anything** to get money to gamble?

> Have you **wondered** whether you have a problem with gambling?

> Has your gambling caused you any **health problems**, including feelings of stress or anxiety?

> Have **other people** criticised your betting or told you that you had a problem with gambling (regardless of whether or not you thought it was true)?

> Has your gambling caused any **financial problems** for you or your household?

> Have you ever felt **guilty** about the way you gamble or what happens when you gamble?

Score your answers like this:

> if you answer 'never' score zero

> 'sometimes' = one point

> 'most of the time' = two

> 'almost always' = three

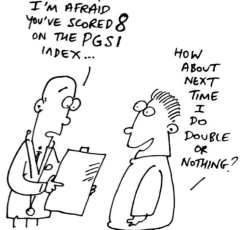

If you have a **score of 3** or more, you're at **moderate risk**. Ask yourself what you can do to regain control of your gambling or whether it might be best to stop.

If you have a **score of 8** or more, you're at **high risk**. Stop gambling. That might not be easy and that's not your fault. These are highly addictive products. Your responsibility is to be honest with yourself about the scale of the problem. If you cannot stop by yourself, get support.

I'M NOT SURE.

You could add other behaviours to the list above.

> Are you **lying** to others about your gambling? Perhaps you're denying you're doing it at all or playing down how much you bet or have lost (or even won).

> Have you ever **stolen** to fund gambling?

> Are you **thinking a lot about gambling** even when not actually doing it?

> Do you feel **restless** or irritable when for whatever reason you are unable to gamble?

> Are you aware that gambling is having **negative effects** on your life, such as in work or relationships, but you carry on anyway?

> Have you **tried to stop** or cut down on gambling but failed to do so?

If you're answering 'yes' to any of these, that is a red flag.

Stop gambling for a month, maybe three months. If you can't do this, you need to stop completely. If you can't stop, seek support.

WHY CAN'T I STOP? I MUST BE A WEAK PERSON.

Addiction is not our fault. It involves genetic, psychological and social factors as well as the brain biology we've already discussed. You haven't got a lot of control over any of those. Remember too that in the particular case of online gambling, the products are deliberately designed to be addictive.

The House of Lords Select Committee on the Gambling Industry found that 60% of gambling industry profits come from 5% of customers. Online it's even worse. Research by the University of Liverpool found that 86% of online profits come from that 5%.

People in this 5% group are addicted or at serious risk of addiction. Pretty soon, if they don't stop, they run out of money, get into debt, turn to crime, wind up in prison or die. All potentially result in dire consequences for their families. This means the industry needs that 5% group to be regularly renewing itself.

You will have seen the slogan 'when the fun stops, stop' on gambling advertising. Perhaps that's the reason you think your inability to stop is your fault.

But, think about it. What does 'when the fun stops, stop' say to someone who doesn't gamble? A child, for example. (Let's not pretend children don't see these ads; they're in the middle of football matches.) The slogan says, quite explicitly, that this activity is fun and that it's something you can stop when you wish to. It's an enticing message disguised as a health warning.

It's not just the gambling industry's apps that know how to pull you in. Their copy-writers are pretty sharp too.

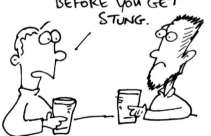

WHEN I STARTED GAMBLING I GOT A BUZZ. SHOULD HAVE REALISED THATS WHAT USUALLY HAPPENS BEFORE YOU GET STUNG.

Nick, 31

As a kid, my gran lived on the coast next door to the arcade. She'd give us coins for the 2p pushers. That was my first gamble. Then it was the fruit machines. By 17, I was playing pool for money.

I had a very comfortable life and went to a private school. But, at the age of 10, I was abused by a teacher. He made me sit on his lap and he'd touch me inappropriately. One day he got arrested. Someone else had complained. I never talked about what had happened to me until 2020. I buried it. I think the way my personality developed was related to that abuse. I had tunnel vision, trying to block everything out. I abused drugs, alcohol and gambling.

I'd win but if I won £5,000, I wanted to win £50,000. Putting a tenner on a horse was pointless to me. My first memory of a problem was aged 18 when I did all my wages in a week-end.

By 21, I was on £38K in London. I didn't understand the value of money. I'd grown up with it. You think you'll always have it. I had one job after another. Always changing and chasing. Nothing was ever good enough. I always wanted the next buzz. I'm probably still the same but now I'm working the 12-step programme to keep me in check.

Smartphones made gambling worse. It was so accessible and it never felt like real money. It's just a number on a screen. I could hold on to real money longer - although not that long. I'd bet on anything in any market - badminton in Croatia, tennis in Spain, anything.

I was constantly betting more money than I had. I was taking out payday loans. (I was in a 12-step meeting once with professional footballers and they were taking out payday loans!) You start lying to borrow money. You cheat and steal. When you're a gambler, you become the best liar in the world.

I'd start a day depositing a £100 into my account and by the end of the day I'd be depositing thousands. Nobody at a bookmakers ever rang me up or intervened.

I was a VIP. Free tickets to events. I won big at a big meeting one year and was invited to all sorts of things - free passes to the best enclosures with £500 free bets. Of course, these bets aren't actually free as you have to bet more than £500 to get them. Once you've lost everything they give you a couple of drinks. It's grooming really. They are exploiting your mental illness. What the gambling sites did to me and what that teacher did to me - they're not a million miles apart, they're both grooming.

Then, as soon as you win big, the sites close your account and say they're doing an 'investigation'. They're just waiting for you to gamble the lot away and eventually you do. It's deliberate. They're ploys to not pay out. I've lost £25,000 in a couple of weeks and they say nothing. I've won big and they've closed my account because of 'money-laundering'. They're not worried about money laundering when you're putting it in. I just don't understand how they can get away with it really. Even to this day, I get emails from gambling sites telling me to reclaim money in my account. It's a lie. There's no money. They want to trick you back into their world.

I went into treatment for drink and drugs in 2020 and that was when I first talked about that teacher. But it was another year or so before I realised I had a problem with gambling. The tell-tale sign is when you start betting in secret.

It was madness. Sheer hell. I had a lot of debt - probably in the region of £400,000, by the end. I was robbing Peter to pay Paul, chasing losses. I had no money to pay what I owed and people started talking.

One night I came clean about my gambling and how I'd robbed people to feed my addictions. If I hadn't, I think I'd have killed myself. I'd already stood at the end of the pier ready to jump off. I had a big social circle but overnight everyone stopped talking to me. People I thought were my mates never rang me again. I was so lonely.

People in the 12-step programme don't judge me. They're my new friendship group. I go to Alcoholics Anonymous and Gambling Anonymous - at least, two meetings a week. Talking about something takes the power away from your thoughts. I'm a completely different person since I met my 12-step sponsor.

People don't understand an addiction that doesn't involve putting something into your body. But writing out a betting slip is such a release. The gambling's been much harder to quit than drinking. There's always that 'what if...?' It's the thrill of the chase.

Now I'm overeating. I'm not even hungry - I just stuff things down. If I like it, I want more. So I have to watch my behaviours all the time. I deal with temptation by going to more meetings, keeping busy and near the phone. I need to work hard in my new business but not so hard I get tired because that leads to problems too. My sobriety is my top priority, even above my partner and child. It's not just about not having a bet, you also need to change.

HOW TO STOP GAMBLING

There is support out there but, first up, some things to do for yourself.

The best way to take a bone off a dog is not to fight with it but to give it something more exciting. What's your something more exciting?

At first, anything you do to replace gambling is good, even scrolling through social media, but eventually you want to replace it with things that are good for you and make you feel good about yourself. The CAN DO challenge (see page 18) can help you find something.

REMOVE TEMPTATIONS

Use blocker apps like GamStop or Gamban to make it harder for you to gamble online.

Are you more likely to bet when you have a drink or when you see particular people or go to particular places? Perhaps you keep taking your phone out and that triggers you. Make sure that you are aware of your personal triggers to gambling and try to avoid them. There might be particular circumstances (home alone), particular times of the week (Saturday), particular times of the year (the Grand National, Wimbledon or whatever).

Stress can be a trigger to addictive behaviours. It may not always be possible to avoid stressful situations, but we can learn to spot our signs of stress such as anger or irritability. (There's more about this in our manual Beat Stress, Feel Better.)

Find ways to relax - exercise, meditation, reading, music, yoga, arts and crafts.

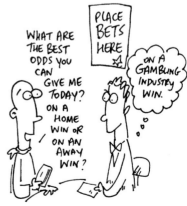

TRY THE 'CAN DO' CHALLENGE

There's plenty we CAN DO to boost our health and find meaning based on the five ways to wellbeing.

The five ways are:

> **Connect** - connect with other people, on or offline, in groups and one-to-one

> **(Be) Active** - move your body - go for a run/walk/swim/dance/etc

> **Notice** - look up, look down, take notice of the environment around you (to do this, turn off your phone for a bit)

> **Discover** - learn something new - this could be something major like taking a course or something everyday like reading a book or watching an instructional video

> **Offer** (or give) - do something for someone else - volunteer, donate, smile.

The easy way to remember the five ways is by the acronym CAN DO. There's so much we CAN DO instead of gambling.

Create your own menu of CAN DO activities. Try to do all five in the course of a week (or a day if you like a challenge). Some activities will tick more than one box. For example, joining a litter pick lets you connect with others, keep active, notice more and offer something to the community.

GO WITH THE FLOW

Whatever your menu, try to include some flow activities. These are activities that you can lose yourself and become totally immersed in. Choose something healthy obviously - don't replace one addiction with another. Find a hobby. Creative activities are particularly good. Hammering away at your guitar, throwing paint at a canvas, dancing madly, singing badly, it's all good.

There's more about the CAN DO approach in our manual Man MOT For The Mind. And if you need some ideas, there are dozens of possible activities in The CAN DO manual. Both manuals are in the Forum's shop. The CAN DO manual is a free PDF download.

TAKE CONTROL OF YOUR MONEY

Do you have a partner or family member who can support you by, for example, looking after your credit cards? Your bank may be able to help by blocking payments to gambling sites or temporarily freezing your card if you're spending a lot.

If you have debts, get advice sooner rather than later from Citizens Advice, National Debtline or a money advice organisation.

PLAN YOUR TIME

Remove the temptation of boredom by planning your days to avoid those thumb-twiddling moments when you might be tempted. (There's some evidence that gamblers are easily bored.)

Set yourself goals, tasks and problems to solve. Get back into old hobbies which you may have lost interest in while gambling.

Take it one day at a time. Invest as much time in your alternative recovery activities as you did in gambling. Accept too, as you'll read in our case studies, that recovery will take time.

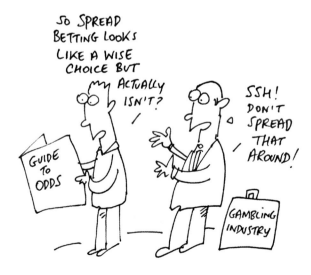

WRITE IT DOWN

Even if you're talking to someone (and especially if you're not), it will help to talk honestly with yourself about what's going on. A proven way to do this is to start a notebook or journal. It sounds like hard work but, in fact, writing for just a few minutes a day can make a difference. If it takes off, you'll soon be writing more. Here are some things you can write about:

> **Gratitude** - experts reckon we need five positive thoughts to overcome a negative one. So everyday, note one thing, big or small, that you're grateful for. Or perhaps two. (It can be a great way to start and end the day.)

> **Achievements** - it's easy to feel negative about yourself when recovering from addiction. Make a note of the good things you've done today at home or work that have helped you or others.

> **Situations** - what situations have made you stressed or angry? Why do you think that is? What did you have control over in the situation? Top of the list might be your reaction. How can you change that in future? You could score situations from 1 to10, depending on how stressful you find them and think about how you plan to deal with them.

> **Your triggers** - what are your triggers to wanting to gamble? Notice them. Perhaps they're related to those stressful situations.

> **Beliefs about yourself** - what do you believe about yourself and why do you think that is? (For example, some of us are told we're stupid or useless in childhood and carry these messages into adulthood as core beliefs about ourselves. Even 'good' parents say these things sometimes and children can take them to heart.)

> **Vision** - what do you want your healthy gambling-free life to be like? Really describe it. Positive visualisation works. You could even add some visuals to your notebook - drawings, images from online or magazines. The value of seeing the positive and accentuating the positive cannot be overemphasised.

It makes a lot of sense to write about all these things. That way you can monitor changes over time. But even if you don't write anything down (it doesn't suit everyone), it is vital that you think about them during your recovery.

BE HONEST WITH YOURSELF

Don't forget the simple fact that, if you gamble, you will lose. Most gamblers lose in the long term and all compulsive ones do.

Your favourite gambling platform is not your friend. They have groomed you and taken your money. Change what you associate with them. Change the face of the brand to someone you loathe. Change their slogan to something negative. Change their logo to something hideous.

TALK TO SOMEONE

Talking with a partner or a trusted friend helps enormously. Support groups and twelve-step groups - see page 25 - can also be useful. As can professional therapists who specialise in this field. It's very useful to be accountable to someone to help keep you on track.

If you really need to talk to someone but don't have anyone around, talk to Samaritans. They're not just for people who feel suicidal and are available 24/7.

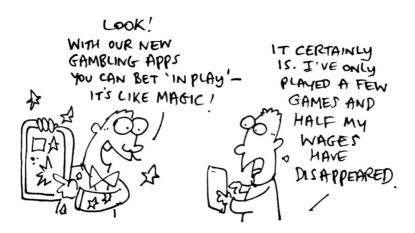

Simon, 41

I was unfortunate enough to grow up in a pub. At the age
of six, I'd steal money from the charity box to play on the fruit machine. I knew
I'd be caught and, when they did catch me, my parents made the terrible
decision of giving me £2 of tokens a week to play on the machines.

I had a building society account and I got keys to that aged 16. I told Mum I
was saving for Uni but I used to take it out and play the machines.

I studied Maths at university and it coincided with the rise of poker and
decent-speed internet. I could use the gambling sites in the computer room.
At first they were genuinely giving money away. Today, there are no 'free' bets.
There were then. But, of course, they were still reeling you in.

I had a student account with an overdraft. The bank noticed the amounts. This
wasn't usual student activity. They closed the account. I did well enough at
Uni but could have done better without the gambling.

In my twenties, I frequently didn't have enough money. I wish I'd realised that
my money could be better used. I was going through bins at one point. I lived
on Weetabix with water.

I was staying up till four and getting up two hours later to go to work. I earned
well which meant I always had a means to cover up what I was doing, pay off
loans and so on. My invoices would clear and an hour later I'd have nothing. I'd
want to gamble on the football on Saturday but lose all my money on the
Monday on something else. I remember, after a job paying me £900 a day,
gambling all my money and sleeping rough because I didn't have the train fare.

I used to pride myself on my ability to get out of the problems my gambling
had created but I hurt so many people on the way. I paid my debts to
everyone except those closest. I remember giving my girlfriend a card I knew
full well wouldn't work and she had to pay for herself.

I could win £700 but if I needed £1000 to pay a bill, that didn't matter. It wasn't
enough. I couldn't stop and I'd lose it. Next morning you realise: that £700
could have been useful. But self-destructive people like me are attracted to
both winning everything and losing everything. For me it was a perfect storm:
I'm either going to win big and make my life better or I'm going to lose big and
get closer to my rock bottom and then I'll get well. Crazy thinking.

It wasn't even about the amount of money. I was as happy if a 10p bet won as a £100 one. It's all about having a bet that's still active, a possibility, something to look forward to. 'Well you never know.'

There are many points of no return but, once you start lying, it's a slippery slope.

I was laying football bets. I set up a gambling syndicate using data and spreadsheets. It worked for a while but it was unsustainable. At the same time, a friend stole a lot of money.

I needed a couple of big loans to cover the hole. I was on my honeymoon with a £50k hole to fill. One night, while my new wife slept next to me, I won £60k on the spin of a slot. I withdrew it, then decided I needed more. Anyway, it was so easy, I reversed my withdrawals and lost it all. My wife had no idea. Lies to cover up lies. It's a miracle she's backed me and we're still together.

July last year was my rock bottom. I considered taking my life. I left home with no money or phone and went missing for five days. I was sleeping rough. Debt was catching up with me. I owed about £100k overall. I'd been offering people double their money to come in on a bet with me and, because I'd made the promise, I'd pay up. I borrowed £5k off one friend to pay someone else double the £2k they'd put in. I hadn't even placed the bet. It was madness.

It was all about keeping face at any cost. It became easier to think about killing myself than having to admit my lies. I was high-functioning, manipulative and very good at keeping up appearances. It's an awful combination. If I hadn't been clever, I wouldn't have been able to get myself into so much trouble.

When I came back, I realised people loved me and your delusions of grandeur don't matter. People who love you, love you as you are. I realised I didn't want to die. All I wanted was a simpler life.

I think now that the happiest times I had were when I had no money at all and couldn't gamble. Now, if I have money, I'm like Frodo with the ring. I don't like it. My wife controls all my money.

I'm always going to be a gambler. I've got to control it. I know what I am, who I need to be with and how to behave. I'm lucky I have someone to support me.

Every addict's story has chapters which could all have the same title: 'my next excuse'. I'd say that, if your gambling is making you lie, hurt people and do things you'll regret when you wake up, get real. There is help but only if you wake up. If you're at the point when you need to win, there is probably something else you should be doing with your money.

WHAT CAN HELP?

THERAPY

The NHS reckons that cognitive behavioural therapy (CBT) is probably the most useful type of therapy for gambling issues. CBT teaches you skills to reduce your urge to gamble and tries to replace unhealthy negative beliefs with healthier positive ones. Family therapy may also help.

MEDICATION

If a mental health challenge such as bipolar disorder, depression or anxiety is part of your compulsive gambling, antidepressants and mood stabilisers may be prescribed. Drugs called narcotic antagonists which are used to treat some drug addictions can also be used in gambling.

TALK TO YOUR GP

Both therapy and medication to help with gambling disorder should be available through the NHS.

If you live in England or Wales, are aged 13 or over and have complex problems related to gambling, you can refer yourself to the National Problem Gambling Clinic in London, which includes the Young Persons' Problem Gambling Clinic.

In England, the NHS also runs three other specialist gambling clinics (the NHS Northern Gambling Service based in Leeds, the NHS Southern Gambling Service near Southampton and the West Midlands Gambling Harm Clinic in Stafford). Talk to your GP.

SELF-HELP GROUPS

Some people find that talking with others with similar issues is helpful and supportive. Gamblers Anonymous brings together men and women who want to do something about their own gambling problem and support others. It is based on similar principles - the twelve steps - to Alcoholics Anonymous. There are also GamAnon support groups for friends and family.

Some of the other organisations listed here also offer self-help groups and forums.

YOUR WORKPLACE

Your employer may offer an employee assistance programme (EAP) which should be free and confidential and may include support for gambling issues.

GAMCARE

GamCare runs the national gambling helpline which is open 24/7 by phone, text chat or WhatsApp. They also run group chats. GamCare can point you towards other sources of advice and support.

GAMBLE AWARE

Formerly known as the National Gambling Support Network, GambleAware brings together organisations across Great Britain who provide free, confidential and personalised support to those experiencing problems with gambling or affected by someone else's gambling.

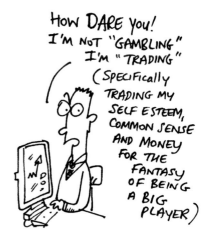

GAMSTOP

Free online self-exclusion tool preventing you from accessing gambling sites (gamstop.co.uk).

CHAPTER ONE

Also for both gamblers and those concerned about them, the Chapter One website explains the causes of gambling harm and where to access the right help, free from gambling industry funding and influence (chapter-one.org).

OTHER USEFUL ORGANISATIONS

> **Gambling With Lives** - a charity set up by families bereaved by gambling-related suicide (run the website Chapter One mentioned above)

> **Big Deal** - provide information, advice and support for young people

> **Gordon Moody** - a charity named after the man who brought Gamblers Anonymous to the UK. Offer residential treatment and an international app in a variety of languages

> **BetKnowMore** - a charity founded and run by people with 'lived experience' of gambling dependency and recovery.

BE AWARE OF INDUSTRY-FUNDED SUPPORT

There are many organisations out there that offer support with the harms caused by gambling. Some receive voluntary funding from the Gambling Commission's licensed operators (ie. the gambling industry). You can see who gets what on the Gambling Commission's website where there is a list of organisations for operator contributions.

While the support you might get from industry-funded organisations may well be helpful, it is unlikely to stress the key role that the industry and their products play in fuelling addiction and is more likely to focus on your responsibility, rather than theirs.

Tom, 34

I'd spend the week looking forward to the high

I only ever bet on football. I loved the game as a kid.
Collected all the stickers. Remembered all the stats. My first bet was aged 17.
I was tall enough to walk into a bookies. But it wasn't a big deal.

Occasionally I'd gamble more than I should have done, but I'd be able to leave
it for months at a time if need be. It became a problem in my late 20s. I
graduated university late and moved to London. I didn't have a well-paid job
and earned less than my friends who'd graduated about five years earlier. I
spent a lot of weekends indoors watching football.

Then I had a big win by my standards - a month's salary or more - which
kick-started it. Wow, that was easy. Why don't I do that again? I used to spend
the week researching and planning my week-end bet - an accumulator over
several games over the course of the week-end.

When you land an accumulator, you get such a strong rush of dopamine. I'd
spend the week looking forward to the high. I was up financially for several
months and didn't see it as a problem. But looking back, I was absent,
distracted and withdrawn the whole time.

I hit a losing streak and started to bet in the week to chase losses, betting on
games I didn't know anything about. Second-division Asian games in the
middle of the night. Gambling took over. Everything around me started
unravelling, over the course of a year or so. Work, my relationship, friendships.
I wasn't putting the time into any of them.

At that point, I didn't link the gambling to my other symptoms. I felt depressed
and anxious. I was not exercising or eating properly. I felt at my lowest when
the gambling session stopped. I'd be full of self-loathing and misery. Now, any
sense of excitement was replaced by fear.

Overall I probably lost about £10-11,000 in the 18 months it was at its worse.
It wasn't nothing but the debt wasn't insurmountable. The damage to my
mental health was far more costly.

Friends would want to go to a match or meet up to watch one, but I wanted to
stay at home alone following the scores online. My partner and I had moved
into our own place and it wasn't good. The gambling industry would claim I
was 'vulnerable' because I was going through a difficult time, but it was the
other way round: I was going through a difficult time because of gambling.

I'd self-exclude from the gambling sites - you had to do them one platform at a time - but I'd always go back and plead in the live chat to have my account reinstated. Nobody at any of the companies ever asked why I'd blocked myself in the first place.

The single most helpful thing

I started to look for help, but there wasn't really anything there. It was about setting financial limits or time limits and I couldn't do that. I felt even worse about myself and very isolated. The message the industry gives is that anyone who wants to stop can stop and I felt a failure because I couldn't. I now know this is not true. Nobody would advise an alcoholic to 'have just one'.

I saw my GP. I described the symptoms. No interest in anything. Couldn't sleep. Could barely get through the day. They asked about drinking but I had to mention gambling. I was prescribed anti-depressants which didn't help. They take so long to kick in.

My relationship was in tatters. We couldn't afford to live by ourselves, so we were stuck together. My girlfriend said we had to talk. She was in tears, packing her bags. I was hardly listening, watching the game on a betting app out of her sight. I remember the game: Manchester United v Everton.

That was my rock bottom. Luckily, I had a friend round the corner who I started spending more time with after my girlfriend left. I told him everything. He helped me realise that gambling was the cause of my problems.

I found the tool GamStop, which is a nationwide self-exclusion tool. You're locked out of every online bookie licensed to operate in the UK. This may have been the single most helpful thing but even then, it took me a few days to click the button. That was the end of online gambling for me. I had a few relapses and went into a bookies, but you have to find one. It didn't get me in the same way as online gambling. Taking out £100 felt like real money compared to credit and debit card betting. Plus all the apps are designed to keep you there. It wasn't same in the bookies, which was not a place I wanted to be in any longer than I had to.

So I stopped, but I hadn't really analysed it. I discussed it with a therapist. It was helpful but she wasn't an expert in addiction. She certainly didn't know anything about gambling.

I carried a lot of self-blame and shame around for a while until I got involved with Gambling With Lives (GWL). I heard about the charity on a podcast. Someone, who is now my colleague, framed it as a mental health problem developed by a malignant industry. It was the first time I'd thought about it that way around. It was like someone had opened the curtains. I began to understand what had been done to me. I got in touch and a couple of months later started working for GWL. Another key point in my recovery.

Addiction to online gambling is not an accident

I now know how dangerous certain gambling products, like online slots and casino games, are. At least in a real casino there are some checks. Online, there are none. The maximum stake on the FOBTs spin machines in bookies were reduced from £100 to £2. You can still lose a lot, of course, but online it's worse. The equivalent online games are uncapped.

Addiction to online gambling is not an accident. It has been done to you. The apps are designed to hook you. The industry will blame you, throwing around words like weak and vulnerable and call you a problem gambler. But you're not the problem, they are.

There are established treatment pathways for drugs and drink, but very little for gambling outside what is provided by the industry itself. Platitudes like 'when the fun stops, stop' will, when you can't stop, just make you feel worse and exacerbate the mental health problem.

We need a statutory levy on gambling industry profits. A levy of 1% would generate about £140 million a year to go towards independent treatment and public health messaging run by the NHS. Currently most third-sector treatment is actually funded by the industry and perpetuates the individual responsibility model, which is so dangerous.

We need to improve education of children too. We wouldn't let the tobacco industry teach children about the dangers of smoking, so why are we letting industry-funded charities teach them about gambling?

We want improved training for GPs and health professionals and third parties like debt advisors. GPs need to ask about gambling as they do about alcohol. At GWL, we're working on developing some materials.

We want an independent ombudsman. Currently, it's cheaper for the industry to continue to take money off addicts while paying the odd measly fine. They need to be forced to change their harmful business model.

We want a ban on gambling advertising as with smoking and an end to VIP schemes. We want sensible, accurate, informative public health messaging. Gambling can seriously damage your health. I know that.

> Tom works for Gambling With Lives, a charity set up by families bereaved by gambling-related suicide.

TAKE CONTROL

There's nothing wrong in principle with putting a bit of money on something. It might spice up a pool game or watching a football match. Betting like this with a mate is unlikely to hurt you. Nor will the occasional lottery ticket or day at the races.

The issue is our ever-present digital devices, the way gambling works in the digital age and the way online technology is being exploited by the industry to part you from both your money and your wellbeing.

There are many drugs that many people choose not to take. They don't do this for moral reasons or because they believe the drugs won't be fun or exciting. They do it because they know the drugs are highly addictive. Whether you think gambling and particularly online gambling is one of those drugs is your choice.

But whatever you do, bear this in mind: however enticing those websites or apps may look, they are not your friends. They are pushers and they want to get you hooked.

Neil, 58

I had an unhealthy relationship with money from the age of six. I remember seeing older guys playing cards and all I saw was the money as they sat in a circle on the street corner. I didn't want it to buy sweets or anything like a normal kid would do; I was strangely magnetically drawn to the money itself. As a kid, I started gambling under the lamp posts playing cards.

Later on, I was openly playing cards in my mum's house during the weekends. My hands were black at times with handling the coins by playing constantly around eight and, on occasions, 24 hours. At school, I decided I was thick, stupid and inadequate after being kept back for another year for Primary 5 and became the class clown from that day on.

At the age of 16, I was already borrowing money to fund my gambling. I was diagnosed with drug-related schizophrenia at age 19 as a result of taking magic mushrooms. I was 21 when I went to prison for theft; again, gambling-related. I thought to myself: how do I change my life? I decided to move away from my home town. I decided to stop gambling. I decided to have my teeth done.

I got counselling for the gambling, but I just told them what they wanted to hear. I'd promise to budget my money, and I'd mean it when I said it, but as soon as the money touched my hand, it was different. I would know the race time of dogs and horses and looking at the clock triggered me to gamble, and that was it, I gambled again, back in the loop!

A woman, the receptionist in the homeless hostel where I stayed, unbeknownst to me, was a member of Alcoholics Anonymous (AA). She asked me if I wanted to stop gambling and I said yes.

She arranged for a member of Gamblers Anonymous (GA) to take me to a meeting that same week. This man drove 20 miles just to collect me to take me to my very first GA meeting. I cried when I read the questions they asked. I thought: how did they get in my head?

I knew I was in the right place but, at that point, I only related to gambling as a financial problem. Although I wasn't educated, I had a Masters degree in how to screw up at gambling. After three months of not gambling, I was, of course, much better off, no financial problem, so I thought I was cured. I stopped going to GA and relapsed.

I went to London with a girlfriend. It didn't work out, but I stayed in England. I travelled in the south of England for twenty years. I was in homeless hostels and sometimes in psychiatric institutions.

All that time I was going to GA, but I was still gambling. I'd sometimes get social security, sometimes work shifts - that was how I survived as a gambler. I did a couple of short prison sentences as well.

By 2000, I was drinking three bottles of cider a day. Constantly topping up. One day, I was coughing up blood and found myself in a detox unit for street homeless. They gave me Librium to come off the alcohol withdrawal but, even then, when people suggested to go to an AA meeting, I thought: I'm not that bad.

It took me another five years before I realized that it was the drink that was making me ill. It was in 2005 that I had my last drink, attended Alcoholics Anonymous and got hit very hard with reality. Gambling and drinking can both take you out of reality. I was 40 years old then.

During that time, there were far more AA meetings than GA and that helped. I got a sponsor to work with the 12 steps. I had been like the Wizard of Oz. I had this big flash, street bravado, swearing and loud. But behind the front, there was a little frightened man behind working the controls.

I knew I had to change. I got myself a Thesaurus. I had to learn the new language and stopped swearing to fit into the real world.

Since then, I've spent 12 years in education. I've gone from level three in English to a diploma. Now I facilitate online courses, and drop-ins for gamblers. I've done talks all over the world, once in a Philippine prison. I've even run the Brighton Marathon. I've got married. I told my mum I loved her for the first time a few years before she passed away.

For me, it was the realization of the feeling of being disconnected to the world at large, and from humanity, that made me stop the addiction. And for a gambler, it's even worse as you have to admit defeat and that's very hard, being competitive.

Through my experience as a therapist, I see problems gamblers have difficulties with: your job's gone, your wife's left, your hygiene, appearance and mental health have all gone down the pan and still you're chasing.

My mum used to say to me: 'who did you think I am, Carnegie?' I didn't know who he was.

> I was like the Wizard of Oz. I had this bravado

But at college, I had to pick someone famous to write about, so I chose him.

As it turns out, Andrew Carnegie was a philanthropist in the early 19th century who built 2,000 libraries as a contribution to society. His works inspired me to invest in myself. This got me into personal development and neuro-linguistic programming. Now I use guided meditations in my work. I rediscovered the magic of simple things like going for a picnic in the forest, dance like no one is looking and sing at the top of your lungs!

For me, with the way the society is set up, people can easily fall into different kinds of addiction, and for gambling, it's way easier to fall into it as you are promised something for nothing. In my journey of recovery, I can still hear the words of my sponsor, 'There is no such thing as failure, only feedback!' and this has guided me well through time.

> Neil is still working on his personal recovery by attending GA and AA meetings regularly, while using his education and lived experience to support other gamblers and affected others as a qualified counsellor.

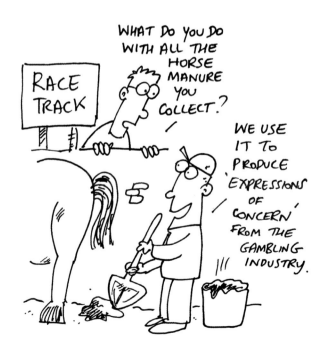

YOUR CHECKLIST

If you gamble, answer the questions on page 12 and score your answers. This page gives you space to record your scores over time and see if they're changing. You can also note how you feel about your score and your gambling.

Answer honestly. If your scores are going up, read this booklet again and take action...

Date:	'PGSI' score	What I think about my gambling right now...